BILLIONAIRE HEALTH SECRETS

DOUGLAS DE BECKER

CONTENTS

PREFACE 3

INTRODUCTION 6

CHAPTER 1 11

    GENETICS 11

CHAPTER 2 31

    FAMILY 31

CHAPTER 3 54

    FRIENDS 54

CHAPTER 4 62

    COURAGE 62

CHAPTER 5 71

    HUMOR 71

CHAPTER 6 79

    INTUITION 79

CHAPTER 7 85

    FOCUS 85

CHAPTER 8 93

    RELATIONSHIP 93

CHAPTER 9 108

    AUTHORITY 108

CHAPTER 10 114

    HEALTH 114

PREFACE

Though many know Gavin better, I knew him first mainly through my imagination, and then through learning if my accurateness of details were correct or not.

My curiosity about my elder brother has always been filled with mostly fantasy, since he was not very present and though I feel both of us did what we could, we were absorbed in a common goal to unlock many secrets of life; time passed us and now we are deep in our life mission and though we are busier than ever, we are now are making time to explore our related-ness, having children of similar ages, and recognizing the opportunities that family gives us that no price can be put upon.

I always made a distinction of Gavin being my "half-brother" along with his sister being my "half-sister", until I simply had to get over the distinction and just call him my brother, like I did every man, friend or relative. Though my distinction was an effort to be honest and exact, it took away from the intimacy of having more family and was extremely awkward all of the time.

In this book I hope to convey Billionaire Health secrets from a perspective of affirming ancient traditions' suggestions and observations. The "authority" of many ancient cultures, were not seen as a personal opinion, but as a learned expertise that was an accumulation of thousands of years of transferred life experience.

Through healthy human relations many common ideas were reached among different groups of people, and some of these still exist today among the ancient cultures that have remained virtually unchanged for thousands of years, such as in the Andes, the Himalayas, and other remote areas of the world. I have personally lived in many of these areas and witnessed differences between those cultures and the western ones, and hope to convey some of the valuable lessons I learned and how a genius such as Gavin, who may not have had the opportunity to travel and live among these people, seems to embody a lot of that wisdom and the health promoting habits that propitiate physical mental and emotional health.

Billionaire Health Secrets thus is not a book about nutrition, herbal medicine, modern supplement hacks, magical - ancient or modern therapeutics, but is about those valuable things money cannot buy, and only perseverance and care can bear the fruit of wisdom that ensures self reliance, honesty, humor, courage and family; the epitome of the fountain of youth.

INTRODUCTION

For most people, billionaire status means tremendous freedom and almost limitless accountability. Though in some ways this is absolutely true in a world built upon economic position, many people who achieve this status have values and ethics that go beyond most hardworking people. My own brother is one of the few billionaires I have heard of and the only one I have had the opportunity to spend time with.

To me, he was my brother, someone who specialized in security and had been the security advisor for Ronald Reagan and some movie stars. I knew very little about him or my sister Chryste, who was so secretive about her career that no one in my family, including Gavin, knew until after she had died.

Some time in my mid-twenties, I called him several times in a year. Almost every time, I received a return call from someone at his company. "Hello, I am calling for Douglas." "Yes, this is Douglas. Who is this?" "I work for Gavin, and he wanted to let you know that he received your message and wanted to make sure that everything was okay." "Yes," I would say, "I was just calling to say hello."

Slowly it began to dawn on me that he was someone very special in our country and the world. Working with movie stars, actresses, and governments wasn't of much interest to me. I had dedicated my life to spiritual practices, seeking out mystics and medicine traditions around the world, and their approach to the riddle of existence. After saturating my life with unusual experiences away from home, I had kids. My focus on developing a practice rooted in ancient medicine practices from the traditions of ancient cultures eventually brought me back to consider my unusual upbringing and my family life, and the mysterious figures of my brother and sister from a different mother, who were raised in a different home than me.

Gavin had an unusual childhood formats, yet unfortunately not too unusual for others. It was full of violence, aggression, and dangerous scenarios, at least where guns, drugs, and money are concerned.

Gavin's focus and mission to reduce violence and protect people was quickly recognized, perhaps because of his unusual photographic memory and exceptional I.Q. He was intelligent, bright, and focused, and was clear in his communication about how he felt, his unique perspective, and opinion; seeded and nourished by his childhood experiences and a drive to change the rise of violence in society.

He told me a story about when he was first invited to speak in front of government officials. They had called him in because of an article they had read, which to them, was an example of someone with great experience and insight in the realm of violence and threat. Little did they know that he wasn't even twenty years old, and this "punk kid," in Gavin's words, was standing in front of some of the most experienced people in world threat assessment, disagreeing with some of their fundamental principles?

Not just opinion but with great reason, he explained why their logic and approach were ineffective and unrealistic. He was quickly appointed as an expert in the field and created a nationwide screening technology to accurately identify violent criminals and thus help to curb the rise of violence. Though his suggestions have not always been welcomed and have sometimes been ignored by the greater powers that be and the agendas that be, he has never wavered from his hard-learned lessons of the power of intuition, accountability, and self-reliance, clearly expressed in the essay "Self-Reliance" by Ralph Waldo Emerson.

In this book, I hope to express with gratitude and admiration how the exposure to such an unusual person has influenced my life and my practice in medicine. This is also my own story and how the idea of protection is a cornerstone of good health, not just from violence, but in an age where the authority of our health is put in the hands of groups with agendas focused on capital gains at best and crippling the self-reliant clarity of one's purpose in "returning to nature," as Emerson would say, at the worst.

CHAPTER 1

GENETICS

The news hit like a tidal wave. My younger brother Brian's voice trembled as he told me his son, Caleb, had passed away. Caleb's short life had been a symphony of struggles and small victories against neurofibromatosis, a cruel disease that marred his body but never his spirit. Reflecting on Caleb's life was a mirror to the trials faced by our family, where resilience was an inherited trait, woven into our genetic tapestry. Brian's life journey was a path lined with thorns. He lost his first 2 wives to the dark abyss of addiction, and the second to a tragic accident sealing his solitude. Their only son was born with a complicated cancer called neurofibromatosis, considered a terminal illness from the very first diagnosis. One of his feet was disabled and turned, and even after many operations to straighten it, the final result because of the cancer was him having to get his foot cut off.

Caleb, their only child, was a beacon of joy despite his relentless battle with tumors that seemed to sprout like malevolent wildflowers. His crippled foot, a testament to the many surgeries, was eventually amputated, a cruel cut in more ways than one. Caleb's optimism, however, was unyielding, his joy infectious. At his funeral, a sea of faces, many who had met him only once, bore testament to the light he had spread. My brother Brian was devastated. It was pretty profound, quite deep, and quite impactful for me and those who were close to Brian.

Brian once asked me to be more present for Caleb. My globetrotting lifestyle, filled with exploration and academic pursuits, had distanced me from family. I regretfully realized too late the depth of their struggles. Caleb's illness was a looming shadow I hadn't fully comprehended. His passing left Brian shattered, and it underscored how I had failed to be the support my brother needed..

Knowing what he was going through, I didn't realize the depth of what he was going through with his son who had a terminal illness. It was known that he would only live so long, and before his teens he passed, my brother was left shell-shocked after several intense occurrences with his job as a policeman, the loss of his wife, and now Caleb.

Caleb's memory lingers, not in the suffering he endured, but in the joy he radiated. He was a quiet child, his questions piercingly profound. He had a habit of ensuring everyone was comfortable before he could relax, his smile a balm to the weary. His spirit was an epitome of compassion, a quality he may had inherited from our lineage, or perhaps just from the knowledge of his health situation.

Our family history is a mosaic of trials, triumphs, and untold sacrifices. Gavin, my older brother, and I often reminisced about our father, whose life was an odyssey of hardship. Growing up during the Great Depression, he lost his father in his youth under harrowing circumstances. Our grandfather's dying words to our father, "Son, I am never going to get better," were a cryptic forewarning. Our father, too young to grasp the finality, couldn't convey his care before his father succumbed to throat cancer.

I reflected upon what a great father, we had all shared.

Our father also lost his father when he was in his youth. Having unresolved arguments and not understanding the communication that had happened, his father pulled him into the room and told him,

"SON, I AM NEVER GOING TO GET BETTER"

As a young boy, my father didn't understand that it meant he was going to die. Not long after, in a private conversation that his mom and dad had, our father overheard his dad speaking with his mom,

"SO WHAT DID HE SAY? DID YOU TELL HIM YOU ARE GOING TO DIE?

Our father said,

"I TOLD HIM I WAS GOING TO DIE AND HE DIDN'T SEEM TO REALLY CARE AT ALL"

Our father felt very confused. He didn't realize that his dad was saying that he was going to die.

And before our father had a chance to clear that up with our grandfather, to let him know that he did care, he passed away from hemorrhage and throat cancer.

Our father's grief was compounded by cleaning the blood from our grandfather's hemorrhage, a macabre task that underscored his early encounter with death. Our mother, too, learned of her father's demise through a tragic news broadcast about a fire. The silent suffering they endured shaped their resilience and, by extension, ours.

My father waited for his mom to come home from the hospital, only to find out that his father had passed away.

Gavin's close adult relationship with my father came later in life, as Gavin was raised by a different family, having a different mother in a very different situation, and there had been a lot of difficulties to overcome.

Reflecting on my father's life, I saw parallels in our family's resilience. Despite the geographical and emotional distances, the bond of shared history and inherent virtues remained unbroken. Honesty, compassion, humor, courage, and self-reliance were our family's bedrock.

My mother had a very similar situation. She was watching television and saw a program on the news talking about a local fire. And as it turned out, they reported that her dad had died on the news. She heard his name reported as one of the fatalities. And that's how she found out that her father had been killed in the fire, waiting for him to come home. He was also very beloved and similar to my younger brother,'s son Caleb. Many people came and only met him once. He was known for his kindness and his generosity.

The importance of being a father and the appreciation of having a father continue to grow inside of me.

I didn't spend much time with my family after I moved from our hometown of Las Vegas when I was about 30. There would be rare holidays that I would come back to visit. I tried to make it more of a point as I got older. Had I known that soon my father would be getting vaccinated and died in a hospital without a single doctor coming to his room, of course, I would have made a point to visit more. Sometimes, we would have significant conversations, and sometimes, the intensity of his losses in life would squeeze him into becoming a mean older man. He was artistic, sensitive, and misunderstood, and his tolerance faded with age.

Just as often, our conversations were short; sometimes, we would also have a brief, small fight. One of the last conversations I had with my father was one of the lessons I still remember.

He called me and was very angry, saying I should call him more if I wanted to get to know him better.

He was very frustrated. Often, he would call, and my voicemail on my phone would be full since he texted infrequently. He would send emails, and I would get most of them, but sometimes I would miss one, and I would typically not get the emails promptly. So he was upset that our communication wasn't strong.

My father's later years were marred by isolation and the ravages of old age. His complex relationship with us, his children, was a blend of profound conversations and sharp conflicts. The pandemic further strained our connection. He was vaccinated, contracted COVID-

19, and despite my brother Gavin's efforts to provide alternative treatments, he succumbed to the illness. It was a poignant reminder of the fragility of life and the importance of presence.

And he was getting old. I had only found out that he had been vaccinated for COVID when I received a call that he had been taken to the hospital a couple of days after receiving the vaccination. Our father became very ill with COVID. And he was scared about going to the hospital and also about receiving treatment in the hospital. And so was trying to ride it out.

A few people couldn't get in touch with him on the phone. They went over to see what was going on. But he didn't open the door. And finally, they got him to answer. He had been sick in bed for three days and was doing poorly. He was very ill, even having difficulty in breathing. So they brought him to the hospital. The hospital immediately started using the protocol that had been part of the popular agenda in responding to the global emergency.

And this protocol was not helping and killed him unnecessarily, as it had killed many.

My brother Gavin flew in a particular doctor from Florida, my father's primary caregiver. And he administered some Ivermectin immediately, and my father started to get better. On the second or third day, he was markedly better, and at that point, the hospital revoked the privilege to have access to Ivermectin and forbade him to receive that treatment. Two days later, he was dead. I later found that the whole time he was in the hospital room, a hospital doctor never once entered the room. Only nurses were there, following the international agenda's protocol.

I was sitting on a plane, getting ready to visit my father. When I got the phone call. The plane was just about to take off when I got the phone call.

I answered the call "Doug!", "Yeah, Brian, what is it?", "Doug he's gone. Dad's dead," I said "What?" "Dad. Dad's dead." This was a somber echo of past losses, the familiar sound in my brother Brian's voice. "Okay. I'll be there in a few hours." I hung up the phone. The plane started to move, and we took off. As the plane ascended, I was left to grapple with a torrent of memories and regrets. My father's death united our fractured family in an unexpected reunion. For the first time in decades, we were all together, our father's legacy reflected in our shared eyes and stories.

And those two hours!

During those hours, I tried to rest my mind and heart and slowly contemplated his life and primarily how I had shown up in his life - with feelings of guilt and justifications of why I hadn't been closer to our father. I marveled at who was present at my father's death. My older brother Hal and Brian, who hadn't spoken hardly for more than two years, even though they lived only a few minutes away. How was it, that on his last day and with his last breath, my father had brought them together.

The next day, I went to my brother Hal's home, where everyone gathered, and was very surprised to see that my brother Gavin was there, too. He brought his wife and kids, and like me, they were only a few hours late from being able to see him before he died. It was the first time I met his wife and his kids, and we all noticed that it was the first time our family was together in 40 years.

Coincidentally, my mother and stepfather were in town. I believed it was close to Mother's Day, and since most of my siblings live in Las Vegas, my mother and stepfather had gone there so that everyone could be together. So there we all were, together.

Family reunion
Very few words were shared about my father.

One of the things I noticed right away was that as I looked into the eyes of my sister and my brothers, I saw how this was now the way that I would be with my father. For the first time, I saw deeply how my father shined through who they were. Although a lot has been uncovered about my lineage through my mother's side, not much is known about my father's side. Only a few details were here and there. But I was curious because of what I had learned about epigenetics.

For me, it is a fantastic experience to see similarities in world views and ways of dealing with situations that are shared through me with my family.

Our father's family's legacy was rich with tales of resilience though thin in details. From our great-great-grandfather's perilous escape during a political upheaval, to our relative who supposedly perished as a decoy for Louis XIV, our lineage is a testament to bravery and sacrifice. The artistic vein ran deep, with our father's parents and their siblings making significant contributions to Broadway and cinema. Our great-aunt, a pioneer in sound healing, and her cousin, a recognized mystic in the Anglican Church, carried the torch of unconventional healing paths and spiritual quests.

There are also stories of our great-grandfather, as a court composer in England, and that is supposedly what created our small "de" in front of our name. Another figure was Joseph de Becker who was a prolific writer on Japanese culture and wrote the first books talking about Japanese culture and legal subjects of Japan in the early 1900s.

Similar to my brother Gavin, Joseph de Becker left England and married a Japanese woman about 100 years before my brother Gavin was born. Gavin did the same and for the same reason of disagreeing with the authority of the government and its position on certain things, particularly regarding the "9/11" event. My brother Gavin moved to Fiji and later married a woman from Japan. It was a very similar story.

My father, my father's mother, and my father's father were all actors on Broadway. My grandmother, Dorothy, was in the longest-ever run of a Broadway play. My father's father, Harold, was in many, many Broadway plays, in addition to many movies including Sherlock Holmes. Many, many movies list my father's sisters as well. One of his sisters was renowned for making the first recordings of sound healing and was a mystic who had the largest Metaphysical Library in the United States at the time. Her cousin was known as the "miracle cool girl" of England and famous for stigmata in the Anglican Church and the healing work she did throughout her life.

I remember both my mother's mother and my father's mother. Both my mother and father didn't have the closest relationship with their moms. My mom's mom came from a royal aristocrat family. My father's mother, I didn't know much about her other than her acting career. She was a very strong, almost German-Irish woman and had a commanding presence. My father always shrank in her presence. Even though their acting family were friends with well established entrepreneurs and wealthy figures at that time, it was only because of their association with the theatre and their friendship with other relatively famous actors and actresses. They would always go to parties and yacht trips with rich people, but they didn't ever have much wealth themselves.

I heard one story about my father's grandfather that I wasn't sure if it was true or not: that he had died, starving to death, and was found on his mattress, and underneath the mattress were hundreds of thousands of dollars. Because of the Great Depression, my father grew up relatively poor. His father did many things to try to make money, and although they had acting gigs, they didn't make much money. My father's father was also on the radio, doing radio voices.

One of the things my father did have was a strong body. After acting and being in some, I think one of the last movies my father was in was National Velvet. My father was very sensitive to classical music and spent his whole life amassing a massive library of all kinds of classical and modern orchestral music and opera. My father started training in gymnastics at a very young age. Although he had a wiry body when he was young, he was solid and became well-known as a tough guy who grew up in New York.

Shortly after, when he was maybe ten years old or something, he moved to Los Angeles. By the time he was a teenager, he had dropped out of high school. He was 15 years old. He heard some classical music playing outside of his classroom. I remember him telling me with a big smile that he had slowly just gotten up in the middle of class and walked out to find where the music was coming from. And he never went back to school after that. He didn't finish high school; instead, he joined the circus. With his gymnastics ability, he was quickly put into the trapeze and immediately given a job that only a young, fearless teen would be willing to do: climb a 300-foot pole and do a one-handed handstand on top of it with no net. He became relatively famous in the circus circuit - in a traveling circus.

And each month he sent most of his money to his mom at home. He didn't need to spend much money while traveling with the circus, nor did he have much time other than gambling a little bit. Each month, he sent most of his money to his mom. When asked since his father had died, he helped her out, and when he came home after being gone for a year or so, two or three years, she had saved all the money he had sent her and returned it to him to help get him started.

As he came home, my father then became very much in love with ballet and started training as a dancer. With his beautiful body and agility, he became good relatively quickly and began incorporating some of his gymnastics work into Adagio, throwing people up in the air and catching them. That's where he met my mother. They created a particular routine, drove a car from the West Coast to the East Coast, and in New York, they bought a one-way boat ticket to go to Europe to try to take their routine and become stars in Europe.

After a couple of months, they ran out of money and almost starved, living with a few other dancers in a small apartment and eating bread and cheese so that they would have cash for dance class. Then someone saw their dance routine and gave them a five-year contract. My mother was a very talented ballet dancer and had received a full scholarship to Juilliard. She never took the scholarship after being threatened by my father to never talk to her again if she was to take the scholarship and go to the Juilliard School of Arts in New York. So instead, they became big stars and travelled through Europe. During this time, all the letters that he wrote to his son, all the communications he had had with his first son, Gavin, and his first daughter, Chryste, were taken by their mom and not given to them. They didn't know what happened; all of a sudden, our dad disappeared. For many years, he wasn't present.

My father came home to see them, and he even went to California to see them, wondering why he had never received any communications from them. He found out that she had not given them any of the letters. She gave all the letters back to him, and they didn't know what had happened until my father's first daughter, Chryste, died.

CHAPTER 2

FAMILY

My father's first son, Gavin, had an unusual upbringing. His household was filled with guns, drugs, and violence. His father, or I should say his stepfather, didn't live there. He rarely visited and was eventually arrested after six successful attempts to hijack a jet to Cuba. Gavin's mother was a drug addict, and the constant fear and emergencies in their home brought him and our sister Chryste very close. This environment gave him a keen sense of danger, heightened his intuition, and required him to be highly aware of any signs of potential violence and threats. Guns, drugs, money disagreements, and dangerous events forced him and his sister to hide until each event passed. He became incredibly adept at recognizing the early signs of danger and potential violence.

Gavin's upbringing unfolded like a tempestuous symphony, where each note carried the weight of his formative years. Born into a realm besieged by the thunderstorms of violence, drugs, and precariousness, he was thrust into the harsh realities of existence before his tender years could fully unfurl. His mother, ensnared in the clutches of addiction, and his stepfather, a shadowy figure of infamy in the criminal underworld, cast a tumultuous shadow over his childhood. Within this cauldron of chaos, Gavin, his younger sister Melissa, and our older sister Chryste, found themselves intertwined in a dance of survival, clinging to each other amidst the tempest, their bond an unwavering beacon of hope in the darkest of nights.

Raised in an environment where danger lurked in the shadows, Gavin honed his senses to a razor's edge, attuning himself to the subtle whispers of intuition that danced upon the winds of uncertainty. These skills, honed in the crucible of necessity, would later blossom into the cornerstone of his success, guiding him through the labyrinthine twists and turns of fate.

One day, he found his mother dead on the floor, the victim of an overdose of sleeping pills. He had to deal with that situation alone. He was immediately adopted into the home of his best friend, while his older sister had already left the house and later became an infamous and secretive member of the Black Panthers. His younger sister Melissa had to be placed in a foster home because there was no room for her in the same house that Gavin moved into. Rosemary Clooney, who took care of Gavin at that point, and made it clear that he had no home and no money, and his sister simply could not move in due to lack of space,

One of the most harrowing chapters of Gavin's youth unfolded with that tragic discovery of his mother's lifeless form, a casualty of the silent assassin known as overdose. This seismic event marked the cataclysmic shift from one epoch of his life to the next, casting him adrift in a sea of grief and uncertainty. In the aftermath of his mother's passing, Gavin found himself thrust into the embrace of the Clooney family, the sanctuary offered by his best friend's kin serving as a fragile raft in the tempest of his sorrow. However, the cruel hand of fate decreed that his sister, Melissa, would be torn asunder from this fragile refuge, consigned to the unforgiving embrace of the foster care system. The agony of separation weighed heavy upon Gavin's shoulders, a burden too heavy for his tender heart to bear.

This was devastating to Gavin. He had to choose between accepting the generosity of his friend's mother and moving in with them or ending up in a foster home waiting for another possible adoption. Yet, in the crucible of adversity, Gavin's resilience burned brightly, a flickering flame of hope amidst the encroaching darkness. He navigated the uncharted waters of his new life with a quiet determination, finding solace and stability in the nurturing embrace of the Clooney clan. This period of transition heralded a profound metamorphosis within Gavin, as he began to refine the rough-hewn edges of his character, forging them into tools honed for the rigors of the world beyond.

His relationship with my father didn't immediately open a welcoming impression for him to move in with our family in Las Vegas. A few years later, he befriended Elizabeth Taylor and moved in with her, becoming a close friend and taking care of her dogs as they travelled around the world. During this time, his remarkable skills of predicting uncomfortable events and remembering specific indications and intuitive senses of potential situations were refined. This won him the confidence of Elizabeth Taylor and many other renowned and high-profile people who later referred him and even became his clients.

He visited us once during this time, in his later teens, a couple of years after his sister Chryste and my father's first son and daughter. I didn't remember them very well from back then—they were older, and I was quite young. But we had a good connection, and I had no idea about Chryste's hidden life. Later, as I grew up, I heard stories about this brother of mine from my father and older sister. He was far busier than I could imagine and worked for high-profile people. I never really spent time with him, yet on a couple of occasions, I visited him with my father at his beautiful house in Los Angeles that Bela Lugosi once owned. Sometimes, we went simply for lunch or a quick visit. I knew almost nothing about what he was doing. I still know very little about his work. And, like everyone else, I knew virtually nothing about what our sister Chryste was doing.

Meanwhile, my own journey unfolded against a backdrop of turmoil and strife. The echoes of my parents' tumultuous relationship reverberated through the corridors of my youth, their battles fueled by the volatile alchemy of alcohol, drugs, and simmering resentment. My father, a figure of boundless passion and fleeting stability, waged war against the demons that haunted his soul, leaving a trail of shattered illusions in his wake. My mother, a stalwart beacon of resilience amidst the storm, struggled to hold the fraying threads of our family together, her spirit battered but unbroken.

My home life became riddled with complications, with my parents falling into alcohol and some drugs and extreme fighting between my mother and father. My father, having an acting background and a very open emotional scope, would sometimes seem to lose his mind, pounding on his chest like a gorilla, completely confused, screaming, and pounding in frustration with the situation at hand.

Amidst the chaos that gripped our household, Gavin's presence was a fleeting yet profound reminder of the ties that bound us together. Though our encounters were sporadic, each interaction left an indelible mark upon my soul, a testament to the enduring power of familial bonds that transcended the vagaries of time and distance.

When I was an infant, my father tried to break into the production business and, for a short time, was producing some shows in Las Vegas. My mother made the costumes and helped him with choreography, and they successfully created a few dance shows. In their dance career, they had performed with acts like Frank Sinatra, B.B. King, and Lawrence Welk. They had a five-year contract to perform in China, but my mother decided to settle down and have kids with or without him.

After their temporary success in producing shows, they needed more money. My dad had an acting background, having been in several movies as a child and some Broadway plays. He got a job as a collector, excelled at collections, and eventually took over. He placed a lien on all the office equipment because they had problems getting paid. When they went out of business, he took all the office equipment home. He eventually got his first license as a private investigator in Las Vegas, where he worked for the next 40 years.

During that time, I eventually had short conversations with Gavin in my dad's office. I ultimately went to work for my father as a private investigator when I was 15. I became busy focusing on my spiritual inquiries after high school and in college. My brother Gavin was not around much, nor was my sister Chryste. Gavin and Chryste had impressed upon me an unresolved sense of family.

The tapestry of my maternal lineage provided a stark contrast to the tumult that engulfed our home, its threads woven with the rich hues of Latino heritage and familial solidarity. Summers spent in the embrace of my great-grandmother and the loving embrace of countless cousins offered a fleeting respite from the storms that raged outside, a sanctuary of warmth and love amidst the chill of uncertainty.

I sometimes visited my mother's family. Her father, her father's mother, and my grandmother were also very loved by everyone. She was the matriarch of the family, having grown up in Guadalajara. She spoke little English and had two sons, one of them being my mother's father, whom I had never met. When their family got together, it felt almost like a ringing sound in my heart—it was very unusual. So many people were very closely related. There were so many cousins, and everyone was very close.

During the summertime, my mother spent many years growing up as a child, sleeping in the same bed with my great-grandmother and five other cousins. They slept in and cuddled and spent weeks or months living with my great-grandmother and great-grandfather. That history was very apparent, and I always noticed how my mother was sad about not being able to pull that together with her own family. Her mother's grandparents were part of one of the wealthiest families in Mexico, owning all the sugar in Mexico and Hawaii. Her father's mother, was a child of another wealthy family in Mexico with an estate so large that took three days on horseback to traverse. After the Mexican Revolution, her family lost everything and settled in California. They had everything and after the revoloution, they had nothing but each other.

My mother was very close to Gavin and Chryste to some extent, although Chryste and her life were rarely discussed—we didn't know much about her. I remember my mom remarking she spoke with an African-American accent from L.A. and had changed her name to Njeri, which means "Warrior" in Swahili. Even Gavin didn't know what Chryste was doing. At the time of her death, he had high-security clearance. His company trained the CIA and FBI, and he was even President Ronald Reagan's security adviser. While he was doing this, she was breaking people out of jail, housing fugitives, and engaging in other activities that the Black Panthers were involved in to advance their human rights cause. Her lifelong partner once joked with me that Gavin was working for the Reagan administration while they were undercover Black Panthers in a band called Reggae Knights. Not even Gavin knew she was involved in that. This was only revealed at her funeral.

Upon losing his sister, Gavin had a few experiences that opened him to a more spiritual dimension. Listening to people speak about her sacrifice and courage for many hours, he gained tremendous admiration for her life and her mission to help the Black Panthers. When I first visited his family in Fiji, I noticed his love and care for the family he created. He had adopted about 12 children from Fiji, becoming responsible for their livelihood and education and sometimes even reuniting them with long-lost family members. They would all agree on who should be adopted. Some of the children had families, and some didn't. But whether they had parents or not, he chose them from the community he lived in in Fiji.

Gavin's journey towards the creation of his own family was a testament to the indomitable spirit that burned within him. After years of tumult and upheaval, he found solace and purpose in the fertile soil of Fiji, where the verdant tendrils of love and compassion took root and flourished. Embracing twelve children from the local community with open arms, Gavin crafted a sanctuary of nurturing and support, where the seeds of knowledge and wisdom were sown with tender care.

His decision to carve out a new life in Fiji was spurred by a profound spiritual awakening, fueled by the haunting strains of church hymns that stirred his soul. Seeking refuge from the ceaseless cacophony of violence that pervaded modern society, Gavin forged a new path, guided by the twin beacons of love and compassion.

I remember when I visited him in Fiji. It was amazing to see what he had created. He had a few servants who were all like a big family. He had moved to Fiji because he was moved to tears listening to beautiful singing at the local church. It was astounding and healing for him, and he found a meaning he had never known before. It was so compelling that he chose to stay and help the community. When he first went to Fiji, he bought property, built a home, and settled there.

Gavin's career in security and personal protection, spanning continents and generations, bore witness to his unmatched expertise and intuition. Yet, amidst the accolades, his heart remained tethered to the memory of our sister Chryste, whose untold sacrifices cast a long shadow over his soul. Her legacy, shrouded in secrecy and sacrifice, served as a silent testament to the enduring power of the human spirit.

The events of 9/11 influenced him to include in his book how his suggestions and the obvious signs had been ignored. When he moved to Fiji, he made an agreement with the village that there would be no television, as he had expressed in several ways how television had been shown to increase violence. There was even a study indicating that violent crimes increased significantly when television was introduced into an area. His profound experiences with violence and danger influenced his opinion about television. He knew from high-level Intel that people could be manipulated, made afraid of things they shouldn't fear, and desensitized and distracted by those things, resulting in vulnerability and a disconnection from their intuitive signals that would inform them of danger. This vulnerability did not exist before the influence of television.

In Fiji, Gavin's life unfolded like a tapestry woven with the threads of love and devotion. His eventual marriage to a Japanese woman and the birth of his own children marked the beginning of a new chapter, where the echoes of his past mingled with the promise of a brighter future. His commitment to family remained unwavering, a beacon of hope in the gathering storm.

These insights became the foundation of his groundbreaking work in security, which he published in his first book, "The Gift of Fear." When I recently visited them, seeing the new family unit he had created and his importance to the family was very moving.

I was saddened to hear him relate the story of how one of his children in Fiji had died during the COVID-19 pandemic. At the time, the opinion of the experts he relied on in his business, were among the most educated and expert in the academic field, and he did not agree with the diagnostic measures, treatment measures, or anything related to the vaccinations that were hastily pushed through, breaking laws and guidelines intended to protect people. The same immunization and treatment killed not only thousands of people worldwide but also our father. In Fiji, his son had cancer, and Gavin tried to fly him to the USA and Australia for treatment, but COVID-19 restrictions prevented it. When he finally found a qualified doctor in India for the appropriate treatment, they sent a helicopter to transfer his son immediately; yet he died before the plane arrived, after many delayed responses and the passage of time in making emergency appointments—denied and died, due to COVID restrictions.

His expertise and insight regarding protection and threats are highly sought after by the most influential people in the world. He manages hundreds of employees who help fulfill his responses to those requests and sometimes deals directly with clients to answer questions that his employees need help answering. This takes up a significant amount of his time. However, he has managed to be fully present with his family, joking, playing, and dedicating quality time to them. In my experience, family has been as essential to him from a young age as it was to our father and mother. I am thrilled that I can slowly create more of a sense of family with a brother who has always been admired by the family I grew up with. He has always been honored and respected.

Throughout our respective journeys, Gavin remained a steadfast beacon of wisdom and guidance, offering invaluable lessons on the importance of family, resilience, and the preciousness of life. Our encounters, though fleeting, served as poignant reminders of the ties that bound us together, transcending the boundaries of blood and kinship.

When I was in my twenties, I reached out to him several times and only received calls back from some employees saying he was swamped but wanted to ensure everything was okay with me. I would respond,

"Yeah, everything is okay." I just wanted to say hello. I never really expected to be very close because of his business, but in the last few years, he has opened many opportunities for communication. I always leave every conversation learning something about life. When I asked him about his Billionaire health secrets he sarcastically said, ""They are secrets."

Since I was very young, he has always "checked" me regarding what's essential in life. I remember being on the beach with him during my recent visit, and he looked so much like my father. I had never seen that much resemblance while we were swimming. He is 69 years old.

He is an older brother my whole family and all my siblings missed and wondered about. At the same time, I accepted the reality that he wasn't there and didn't know why. He reminded me so much of my father and looks like him. I watched him spend long moments with my kids, speaking to them, asking them questions, and learning about their lives. I was moved when he texted me that he was very impressed with the life I had given my daughters. In that text later that day, he said, "It's impressive how you've lived and raised these fine kids. They're awesome and have had so many amazing experiences - with much respect and love."

Wow, I felt honored by his life experience to hear something like that. My sense of family is also powerful at my core. Knowing that part of that sentiment comes from my father makes me appreciate his encouragement in what I do and think. I had a hard time receiving his appreciation and respect, and I feel I have lots of growing to do to unravel why that is difficult for me. Gavin's children were so intelligent, skilled, and free.

When COVID came to where they lived, everyone was required to wear masks. He refused to go along with the authority that said they should wear masks, pulled his kids out of school, and created a home-school, which he shared with other families that agreed that wearing masks made no sense. Today, Gavin has close relations with my siblings. I deeply regret not going to my sister Chryste's funeral, where I could have met many more of her close friends and those who adored and appreciated her. I understand the whole scope of emotions that having a family has allowed me to feel. I'm not hard on myself and don't see life as if it should have happened differently. But I honor whatever sensations I have about how I feel about an event. How I think about that event may change as I get older. I'm still learning more from Gavin every time I interact with him about the preciousness of life and our experiences and feelings.

When I was first at his home in Fiji and became excited about something to share, I started telling him about a particular unusual fact, and he stopped me halfway and said, "No! Your emotions, your experiences, your feelings, I'm all about that. But this type of thing I can look up on the internet if I'm interested in that." Feeling very humbled again, I went back to eating. I started talking again, excited about another fact I thought he would appreciate and be interested in, and after just a few words or a few sentences, he put up his hand and said, "No!" Then he repeated, "No, No."

Then he began to tell me, "When I was young, because of my remarkable intelligence and photographic memory, I often had the opportunity to impress people by sharing random facts and things I had memorized and learned. And though I may have impressed them, I quickly learned that sharing facts and figures created more distance than closeness." (Gavin memorized all of Shakespeare by the time he was 16.) To this day, I still struggle with fumbling over sharing facts and figures. I still need to improve my habit of speaking too much data, something I'm excited about. I do my best to hold on to what he told me, which is still as pertinent in my life today as it was then.

What are my experiences? How do I feel? What are my emotions? Share these things to create deeper connections and nourish the meaning in everyone's life. This is definitely something I do with my children often. I also do this with other loved ones—share how I feel about something and what I experienced. I hope it helps to create a closer family situation in my life.

As I reflect upon the tapestry of our lives, I am reminded of the enduring power of familial bonds that weave their way through the fabric of existence, binding us together in a shared journey of love and resilience. Gavin's odyssey, from the depths of despair to the heights of fulfillment, is a testament to the transformative power of love and the enduring strength of the human spirit. And a key to a long and healthy life.

CHAPTER 3

FRIENDS

As I grew up, I kept hearing about Gavin's amazing life and his friends. He had many celebrity friends, some even romantic. Carrie Fisher, Rosemary and George Clooney, Ronald Reagan, Elizabeth Taylor, Alanis Morissette, Oprah Winfrey, George Lucas, and Robert Kennedy were all his good friends. On my father's side of the family, which had a history of actors and actresses, the names of great directors, actors, and actresses were well known, except to me. I didn't pay much attention to that, but my older siblings did. They would tell me how important some of these people were in the entertainment industry and how

Gavin was friends with them all. Many of these people were also his clients.

As I have grown older, I have come to know of a lot of his clients, mostly from blatant news where I hear about them. For most of my life, I pursued knowledge and spiritual experience, and I never really tried to create a lot of business. I usually just got by, and when I got married and had kids, my focus shifted to financial stability. I had lots of superficial friends because I had a lot of free time, and as I became less available to others, I appreciated how I had some really good friends.

Recently, as I was sitting on the beach with Gavin in Maui, we spoke about the direction of the current government both at the United States federal level, the world economic agenda, and medicine control level, and he told me what he saw and felt regarding the future.

"The worst scenario—a science fiction movie, the worst you can imagine." He had said that to me before, when our father had died, and he was informing us about some of the things that had happened regarding censorship and the efforts to keep experimental, unapproved vaccinations in use and circulation for an unknown sickness that was very questionable, yet not allowed to be questioned.

He told us how a movie had been wiped off of a hard drive of a U.S. movie producer's computer by the British Secret Service, as if our secret service had done it, it would have been illegal. He said matter-of-factly that based on what he had seen and knew, censorship and manipulation of public opinion had been going on for some time.

"This is a rare era where there are collective groups making decisions for the public. For thousands of years, very few people have controlled most of everything, and everyone. This current situation is rare, and the experiment could easily be at its end."

Knowing this, I once asked him, "Would you protect anyone?" For my readers who don't already know, Gavin's business is the top authority on world threat assessment. His company trains "Protectors," who are those rare and skilled warrior/secret agent types who make sure their client does not get assassinated. They usually have military backgrounds—highly trained special force officers, who often seek a position in his company after or when they are done with the military. The Protectors act like what we would call bodyguards; however, they receive unusual training that my brother created. The training includes perhaps the most advanced intuitive training in the world. Thus, knowing what decisions to make, how to make them, when to act, and how to respond to concerns are all part of his unique training that has permitted the survival of the top people in entertainment and politics to avoid violence and, in many cases, death. Most of his work he calls "anti-assassination" work.

Another part of his work is about protecting people's privacy about their relationships, their dramas, and even the events around their deaths, as with his friend George Harrison, whom he was with when he died, and assisted in keeping his body out of the public eye. Can you imagine? Stuffing one of your best friends into a car and pretending he was actually put into an ambulance instead, so that the press didn't get photos of his dead body. This is what my brother did. It's my impression that many of his clients either already are or soon become his friends.

When I went to Fiji, courtesy of a honeymoon wedding gift for my wife and me, we were introduced to two of his good friends. One was General Rombuka, who had overthrown the government in Fiji from the Indian-based government and replaced it with Fijian people. The other was a Green Beret who was known throughout the USA as the person who psychologically prepared soldiers and police to kill. As it turns out, killing wasn't a natural thing for people; soldiers had a difficult time killing people, and both police and soldiers frequently experience many psychological issues arising from concealing everything they internally thought about contemplating the killing of other people. He was very against television and video war games that were allowed to be shared publicly and secretly used to identify good potential soldiers by the military.

Because my brother was also against television due to its potential to increase violent crimes, they both became the best of friends. So, back to the question of whether he would work for anyone. His answer to me was generally yes. He told me that if he discriminated who qualified and who didn't qualify for his protection, he would become everything he most wanted to protect people from. However, with a new exception: Mark Zuckerberg's allowance of privacy and personal profiling to become widespread and monetized was somewhere that my brother felt he had to draw the line.

Though Gavin has many friends, I would say that his family takes priority, as most loving parents do. Gavin spoke about how smaller governments and states made more sense because larger countries were always vulnerable to more corruption—governing and controlling large areas and amounts of people. He felt that part of the broken medical paradigm had its roots in a predictable outcome of large government. I remarked on the idea of limiting influence and exposure with the word "ISOLATION." I said that another outcome that could happen would be isolation. The second time I said the word, he told me that word bothered him. He suggested that what I meant to say was "INSULATION," not isolation.

Insulation could be achieved with a small group of friends that were intimate and close. It fulfilled the human needs of connection but also provided a way to not be so influenced by a society that perhaps didn't have the best intentions for family, personal success, freedom, and power. I asked him about freedom of speech, and he asked me, "Do we even have that now?" I said, "...you mean everything that is censored by public media like news, etc.?" And he said, "That's definitely one expression of that, but even on a more basic level, don't we already censor ourselves from saying things that are inappropriate?"

As a friend of Robert Kennedy Jr. and the initial finance source for his presidential election, he told me that when he was asked for help, he helped not because he thought it would make a big difference. He believed that the government-dominant agenda was very much in an advanced condition. Kennedy told him that though that may be the case, "We still should try." "I lent him the money because he is a friend of mine, not because of the politics."

CHAPTER 4

COURAGE

Courageous acts run through the father's side of my family. My younger brother became a police officer when he was 17 and went undercover in many life-threatening and dangerous situations. My older brother, Hal, dropped out of high school and became a stuntman in Vegas shows for a while. Then, he pursued an acting and music career in Los Angeles, CA. That takes guts.

One of the things that make someone courageous is the honesty to admit when they're afraid. Being strong enough to acknowledge fear and still move forward is courageous. See my brother Gavin's best-selling book, *"The Gift of Fear"*, where he talks about how fear informs us when we're in danger. Real courage is the act of honestly admitting that the outcome of what you may be doing may not be so great. When there's clarity and honesty in your fear and you make the decision to move forward, you're being courageous.

In Ralph Waldo Emerson's book *"Self-Reliance"*, he emphasizes trusting ourselves and listening to our inner voice, defined as intuition. This is not conformity to social expectations, which is actually the biggest obstacle to self-reliance. Being prepared and willing to go against the grain of popular opinion in order to follow intuition is what makes one great. Trusting ourselves over others' beliefs allows us to offer our real gift.

I've seen that over and over with my brother Gavin. He has consistently responded in ways that were not expected, and over time, I have come to see his authenticity as one of his greatest qualities. I remember a story my younger brother told me when he reached out to Gavin for help in a financial situation. Gavin responded with an email, "Hello, nice hearing from you. Regarding the money, the answer is no." He wrote, "many things we think are valuable in life, really aren't that valuable. Our breath, however is, and is the most valuable thing we have, yet we hardly ever think about it until our last one. And we are all over that one." All of us had little interactions with Gavin when we were younger and heard these stories. We were all influenced and often surprised by what he would say and where he would be coming from.

The courage to say what needs to be said and to be authentic has been a great challenge for me. Often when I've said what needs to be said, I've faced backlash and felt bad for speaking up. However, as I have grown older, I have noticed how much people appreciate it when I'm honest and say what's really on my heart. One of two things happens: either I realize that what I was thinking was wrong, or the person I'm speaking to is surprised and grows from the experience, appreciating my willingness to share my thoughts. We often think of courage in terms of actions and what we do, but the courage to look and be curious about how we really feel about something, and then the courage to speak or act when that needs to happen, is also important. Some of my best friends and I have had strong pushbacks from each other in the beginning, and later, after we've realized that we're both honest, authentic, and willing to say what's on our minds, the level of trust goes up quite a bit.

I can see how this little book *"Self-Reliance"* has really influenced my brother, Gavin. As Emerson says, social arenas such as religion, which fears creativity; culture, which devalues individualism; the arts, which teach only to imitate; and society, which falsely values so-called progress—all need self-reliant individuals. Ultimately, his purpose is to get people excited about nature.

Gavin knew that he did not like violence. He stayed close to his life experience, became the greatest friend to himself in trust, and took what he had learned and offered that message consistently, as he does even today. He created the most commonly used technology to screen for potential violence, and as a result, has made the world a safer place with less violence. Understanding how to keep peace in the world was the result of a positive integration of Gavin's early life experience.

Each of our past personal stories, even the most terrible and ugliest, has resulted in the best and most valuable things we do today. Of course, our victories and our wonderful experiences create an elaboration of ourselves and influence what we do in a positive way. But what we do stands on the events and situations that make us who we are. Those events that make us who we are have the power to touch the lives of others and deliver transformation in a similar way that transformed us.

How do we become transformed by our experience? I call this now WHO. Why are we sick? How do we heal?

How do we become transformed by our experience?

I call this the new W.H.O.

Why are we sick?

How do we heal?

Overcome Obstacles.

The question, "Why we are sick?" is a natural result of honesty and courage.

The question, "How do we heal? " is a natural result of accountability. We are accountable for finding a source of helpful information that is in alignment with out life, and has been proven successful for thousands of years. Humans have lived in communities for well over 5,000 years.

To overcome our obstacles, we need to understand that <u>why</u> we are sick is a natural result of honesty and courage. <u>How</u> we heal is a natural result of accountability. We are accountable for finding a source of helpful information that aligns with our life and has been proven successful for thousands of years. Humans have lived in communities for well over 5,000 years. We didn't just pop up a few hundred years ago. They were able to thrive and build immense civilizations, and had at least a sufficient level of physical health that accounted for their success. Egyptian civilization thrived for thousands of years, and Indian civilization thrived for thousands of years.

We are only currently learning about the immensity of the civilizations in Mexico, which was recently discovered to be ten times as large and developed as we had ever thought. All over the world, there have been long-lasting civilizations. Learning about how to keep ourselves healthy is not something that we were taught is our responsibility. The only instructions given were how to eat well, and this was regardless of what our body was like. We placed the responsibility for our health on the medical authorities. However, the current collective modern medical authorities have failed in establishing any guidelines or tools to provide health and preventative measures that protect that health.

I have seen how many remaining indigenous people and some of what's left of their immense cultures live. It's not always comfortable and not always easy. In the past, I was often relieved to feel the natural presence of the elements and the hard truth of survival that the people lived so closely to. But after some time, I would feel exhausted and certain kind of stress and would want to return to my comfortable life.

Stress was a big deal to the indigenous people. It was an experience and affirmation of life itself. Integrating that stress and making it part of your strength is a new way of looking at stress for most of the older current paradigms. Yet this integration can make us stronger, and we can transfer it through ceremony, dance, music, festival and holiday celebrations, and theatrical participations. Our relationship to each other benefits from developing different kinds of circumstances. Ideally, we do not hurt each other along the way, and when we "play" together, we can see things in a different way.

I was really shocked to discover that Gavin's kids could play chess so well. According to one of them, the youngest has been playing chess since he was three years old. They also showed me amazing sleight-of-hand and mathematical card tricks, most of which I could not possibly explain

CHAPTER 5

HUMOR

One of the craziest things is that when I was younger, it was obvious that Gavin was really anti-drugs. If you have followed his work, you probably know that his mother was a heroin addict and died of an overdose of sleeping pills. He was responsible for what he thought was giving her medicine in the morning, only to find out later that he was giving her drugs. All the violence and situations that he and his sister were involved in while trying to survive were such a shit show that he was very anti-drugs. He had no reference that there was any kind of positive thing about that. However, through his friends who were successful, focused, and spiritual, Gavin came to understand the universality of spirituality. He really had distaste for authority of any kind. At some point in his life, it was obvious to him that he needed to get some help to keep moving forward. He had all kinds of issues mentally and emotionally because of all the traumas he had been through. And although they may have been subtle, he obviously was not happy about how that was affecting his life.

Though I haven't spoken to him about any of his trauma stuff, I do know that, in his opinion, working with traditional psychedelic medicines was valuable. Eventually, he even co-authored a book about ketamine, writing the introduction of the book about ketamine. So his perspective on drugs seemed to be more specific about certain addictive substances and activities rather than just a dogmatic opinion about anything that shifted consciousness.

"In general," Gavin told me one day as we were in the fresh breeze blowing through the open-aired Fijian home of his living room, "the one thing that all cultures agreed on, the one thing that all modern governments agreed on throughout history is, no psychedelics."

So, this thing that Gavin told me surprised me a lot. Another time, 18 years later, while I was sitting at the dinner table and in front of my kids, he asked me if I had ever done Ayahuasca. Perhaps he'd forgotten because I had told him that when I had visited him in Fiji that day, he shared his views about the position most governments had.

So it was at the dinner table, at a restaurant, with the kids. Since I had brought this up several times before, because my kids' mom was spending a lot of repeated time participating in these kinds of ceremonies, I had no inhibition. With my kids, I have been brutally honest about all my drug adventures, cannabis growing, and all the drama, highs, and lows of the entire subculture, including broken families and failed attempts to hold onto money. Of course, I've also shared my perspective from living for years among several different indigenous cultures on four continents.

I said, "Yes, I have tried Ayahuasca." I told him my opinion of it. I told him, "I'm pretty anti-psychedelics in general, pretty anti the use of plant teacher medicine, even though I consider them to be very sacred." "In spending time with traditional indigenous people," I told him, "I had found that they weren't really consuming these medicines in general. With rare exceptions, they actually considered them very special medicine and they weren't really consuming them like Westerners do - in a consumerist culture, where more is better and relaxing in those realms were not really valued as a constant habitual pastime. It's like consumerism, where it's just something else to consume. So many cultures have these medicines in them, so many kinds a lot of people have never heard of. They know about them, yet in many traditional cultures, the people of the culture may not even try them in their whole life, or maybe they do it once secretly, somehow."

But it's not something that they're selling to Westerners to have a ceremony with them. It's just not part of indigenous culture's life in general, although there are definitely some exceptions in some cultures. For instance, in at least one Amazon culture, everybody does some Ayahuasca together, but only up until they're about 10 years old, and then they stop and normally do not use it again. So it's only when they're very young. In a couple of cultures that mixed with Christian and African religions, they might do Ayahuasca every day as a kind of cult with their founder from a little more than a hundred years ago. But this is an extremely rare occurrence. It was and is still traditionally used for mental and emotional cleansing and to treat mental disorders. I told him, "I find that usually traditional people use it to cure mental disorders where other therapies and herbal cures have failed. Yet in the Western consumer culture, it seems to be overused until it creates mental disorders." "So," Gavin replied to me, "It doesn't sound like you're really anti-plant medicines; it sounds like you are anti-American culture."

"In Tibet," I told him, "Psychedelic mushrooms are known, but traditionally the use has been to give them to someone who disbelieves or doubts the wide scope of healing and harmony that their Tibetan culture has offered, and all the mystic ideas about the nature of our quantum reality. Once they use the sacred mushroom, they no longer have doubts that there is a great treasure in their culture, and the logic of building strength to calm the mind and heart, and exemplify kindness at every golden opportunity."

If you are someone that sees things as they are, everything is very serious. The situation of the world is terrible in so many ways. For someone whose job it is to have awareness about real threats, one can only imagine the impact and seriousness of the considerations. As well as getting informed in unconventional ways (meaning apart from the mainstream story of reality that is generally fabricated by big companies and pharmaceutical agendas).

Humor is only for someone who's honest and perceptive about how serious things are. That one can be funny, sarcasm, and the ability to laugh at what is doesn't happen much in someone that doesn't take someone's instinct seriously. I always grew up with a lot of humor. My family, my father's family was very, very funny, and so was my mother's family. They would laugh and laugh and laugh. One of the things I enjoyed most in my experiences with Gavin was that his sarcasm was so good.

So, funny. Not growing up with Gavin really made it refreshing to see how he had the same kind of humor. Very funny and how seriously we took many things as well. I would say for anyone that knows him, they would probably say one of his biggest qualities is that he's a funny guy.

CHAPTER 6

INTUITION

"Having a sense of when you're in danger," as Gavin has consistently said, "is a natural instinct, like when you have to go to the bathroom." He never speaks without a reason. For example, you might have a sense that you left the burner on the stove, so you turn around the car, go back, and see that the burner was turned off. The question is, was that signal without any reason? Based on statistical data gathered over many years by Gavin's company, there has always been a reason for the intuition to have given a message to someone when they followed it. It protected their life. Gavin has interviewed thousands of people, mostly women who had almost been raped or killed or both. He investigated the factors that saved their lives and the events that led up to their decisions. Where did that information come from? What drove them to make the choices they made?

Another example Gavin told me was when you have to go to the bathroom. You feel something in your gut that moves you to the point where you know you have to go, so you go to the bathroom. There's no question. In the same way, real intuition speaks to us clearly. However, due to what we've been told and the authority we give to sources of information, we question our intuition. According to Gavin, this is unique in nature because no animal in nature is surprised that they're in danger. They have signals they pay attention to all the time and they respond to them, having a heightened sense compared to what we would consider a normal response to intuition.

In traditional medicine, we talk about how our body tells us what to do. We make decisions on what to eat and what to drink. The more imbalanced we become the more wrong choices we make. We start to feel driven to eat more sweet things when we shouldn't be eating sweet. We feel driven to eat more spicy things when we shouldn't. When someone offers us something that would bring our body more into balance and health, we reject it. This is almost verbatim what it says in the traditional texts of "Sowa Rigpa," which is literally the "healing science". Sowa Rigpa is a combination of Egyptian, Greek, Indian, Chinese, and very ancient folk medicine from Afghanistan, all the way up to Siberia and into Mongolia.

When we're experiencing options, our decisions are coming from someplace. That someplace can be the resource of what we've been told and what we've learned. That resource can also be the feeling of more relief based on how we feel. Choosing something that leads us to greater moments of alignment with health is a skill that's developed simply because our nature is to take authority as our safest and most productive source of information. This resource of authority, perhaps originally our parents or even more originally our senses, tells us what to do. When something is hot, we reject it. When something is cold, we want it to be warm. Accidentally sticking your hand in the fire, you pull it back and know that it becomes warm.

This is all direct experience based on how we prefer to feel—peace, calmness, happiness, and a certain level of enthusiasm and creativity that fill our lives with resources we can draw upon. These definitely come from our intrinsic way of interpreting what's helpful and what's not. As imbalances grow, the tendency to reach for something that will just propagate the same dysfunction in our system increases as we get more and more out of balance. If this translates into our human experience and development through life, then the more we get convinced of what gives us a deeper sense of meaning, connection, and relaxation, and what gives us the kind of enthusiasm and stimulation that nourishes us, it becomes a matter of opinion. That opinion in our interpretation is directly related to the society we live in. We're convinced we should have a certain level of wealth, energy, skills in communication, and ability to connect with others.

The problem with this social pinnacle from a traditional medicine standpoint is that we're all different. Some of us have a genetic disposition that makes it very difficult for us to compensate for sweet tastes. We become sweeter and sweeter, eat more sweets, and are drawn to more sweets, becoming very sweet people. Other people are born very hot-tempered, driven, aggressive, and clear about what they need to get done and will get done. They're very spicy people and like their spicy hot food. The recommendation for the sweet person isn't going to be the same as the recommendation for the spicy person. In a society that idolizes one kind of person, one kind of experience, that's going to make it much harder for a whole group of people. The dynamic of expression will become exaggerated. For one kind of person who aligns with the society and can do what the society says is the correct and beneficial activity to create the desired result, society will decrease the value of the other person. That person will have an extra hard time coping with his inability to show up the way society says he should.

Thus, when the fiery person is offered something sweet, he'll reject it. When the sweet person is offered something sweet, they will have a hard time rejecting it and feel terrible about receiving it. They will know that they should be more hot-tempered but will feel intrinsically that they should eat more sweets. This has created quite a mix-up in a society where being driven and productive is glorified over being compassionate and lazy.

CHAPTER 7

FOCUS

In martial arts, a certain kind of focus develops over time. It's not just narrow and pinpointed; it is flexible and strategic. There is flexibility in terms of the senses, where the dominance of one sense becomes more equalized with the dominance of other senses. For instance, vision becomes less pinpointed in front and the peripheral vision becomes enhanced. I would say that my experience in working with successful people is very similar to my experience in a fighting situation using martial arts. As my mentor Clint Arthur has said, he learned at Wharton Business School, "A businessman is always looking back and forth and up and down and always aware of every possible opportunity."

I've noticed that successful individuals I've been with have a lot on their minds. It's not just thinking; they are metabolizing their experience or their strategies, similar to playing chess. A person might be looking at one thing but thinking of several things. He's considering the potential moves of the other, how many moves they have, and the possible outcomes for his next move. This strategizing is something I've sensed in many interactions with Gavin. His love and intention have been obvious in his strategy to empower and challenge me and the decisions and convictions I've made.

I had waited many decades to muster up the courage to ask why Gavin had joined our family when his mother died, it was never really asked by anyone as far as I knew. My father once said that he felt he should have offered his son to come live with him, his second wife(my mom), and his second set of kids. I perceived that he had felt a little regretful and sad that he hadn't actually welcomed Gavin into our home more. The passing of Gavin's mother had left me with thoughts that maybe it would have created stress in our family, that my mother might have had issues, or that perhaps because of the drugs and money issues of his stepfather and friends of his mom, it might have created some problems. I didn't really know, and I felt it was a very sensitive subject that I shouldn't ask about. I just put it to the side; it was never a huge conversation in our family. You know, my sister had a hard time accepting that she had brothers to begin with. At maybe four or five years old, she had made a recording for my mother's mother about how everything was, and my mother encouraged her, during the recording, to tell her grandmother about her new brothers. But my sister said, "Brothers? I have sisters." She hadn't fully accepted that she had brothers, and maybe that was somehow part of the complexity of decisions.

During those days, my sister had very unusual psychic phenomena happening. She would know what somebody was going to say a few moments before they said it. She would comment on whom my mom would be seeing when she went out, and she would comment on what somebody would be saying in a few moments. Knowing so much definitely caused a lot of unusual stress for her. She eventually developed a nodule in her neck that had to be surgically removed, and they said it had something to do with ancient gill formations in the body. So, yeah, after decades of seeing him, even when I saw him during the honeymoon time that I had with my wife at his place in Fiji, I was unable to really drop in and talk to him, even though he mentioned that I should ask if I ever wondered why. I said, "Not really." The truth was I didn't really know too much. All I knew was that I had this brother that he came and visited once or twice at the house, and I remember swimming in the pool with him, was nothing too much to elaborate on. By the time Gavin got busy in his business, he was very, very busy, and we had very little interaction with him.

So I decided to ask him. It took me a couple of months—maybe about a month to begin to call him and then two or three weeks before I could get him on the phone. When I asked him, he told me the situation, what had occurred, and how it was a very effortless process to go into his friend's family's house. With his best friend, since he was always hanging out with him anyway. So it was very simple. The story I had was mixed with another story and was very, very different. Gavin had some confusing understanding of the absence of my father when he and my mother were dancing in Europe, and no communications were being allowed by Gavin's mother. So it wasn't a huge thing for him to just go ahead and move into a different house. In fact, years later after our sister Chryste's funeral, my father would give Gavin all the letters that

Gavin's mom had returned to him. Chryste died not knowing that my father had actually written several times, and had actually been persistently trying to make contact while he and my mother were in Europe traveling and performing.

That conversation was very impactful, and I felt at liberty to explain to him why I hadn't fully understood the invitation to come visit him. When I explained why, he fully understood and extended the invitation again. He said, "Just let me know when the time is right." I told him that this weekend would be good, and he said that worked out great. Four or five days later, we were on a plane to visit him.

We were given directions to his place—the gate number, drove up to the gate, put the number in, drove up to a second gate, and there was someone on the intercom who spoke to us and allowed us to come in. I had been given the instructions on how to get in by someone named Dustin, who I thought was an employee but later found out he was the son of Gavin's younger sister, so actually a relative. We drove up to the house, unpacked our things, relaxed, and were given an invitation to have dinner if we wanted, although it was kind of late. We went to a restaurant to meet with Gavin. Entering the restaurant, it was obvious it was a good restaurant because so many people were there—it was packed. There was a lot of speaking; Gavin stood up, walked towards us, and we said our hellos and sat down. We were joined not just by Gavin but by his whole family—his wife and two kids. We didn't really eat because we had already had dinner, but eventually had some dessert and great conversation.

One of the first things Gavin told me was in response to when I commented on the restaurant, he said, "Yeah, this is my last time here." It was also his first time here. The reason was because the sound of the people speaking was so loud. The reverberation of the walls—they had no curtains or anything to dampen the sound. It became a big distraction throughout every one of our conversations.

The next day, we went to see the beach and ocean and swam—myself, and my two daughters. We were invited the next day to visit the school that Gavin had created, a kind of home-school that several kids attend. We spent a little more time with his kids, and I suggested teaching a class, which I ended up doing a few days later on basic ancient medicine principles. I also met Chryste's grandchild, who is a beautiful black man with green eyes, and his beautiful fiancée. They both warmly welcomed us. That's when I found out that Dustin, who drove up as well, was the child of Gavin's younger sister. We stood there and made some comments about different relatives, and there was an amazing sense of family that I hadn't had since I was young. When I was younger, we spent more time with my mother's family—my uncles, aunts, cousins, nieces, and nephews.

CHAPTER 8

RELATIONSHIP

One night, while I was living in our house on Shadow Lane in Las Vegas, during a time when I was doing an average of one to three hours of an intensive meditation every morning and evening, I heard a knock at the door. It was at least 10 PM, and I lived on a street that didn't see much action or activity. So it was pretty unusual to receive a knock on the door that late. It was very dark outside, and to knock on our door someone had to first open an outside gate and then walk the path alongside our pool. Being in an elevated mood from my meditation and the serenity of my simple life, I opened the door and found in front of me, standing there in the shadows, a tall, thin black man.

One of his arms, his left arm, was shriveled up and hung at his side, unusable and about half the size of his other arm. He said, "Hello." I forget what his name was. He said, "I've come because I need some help. I had polio when I was a child, and that's why my arm is like this. I'm trying to get a job at a restaurant, but I need a health card. I'm wondering if I can borrow $20 to get my health card. I promise I'll bring you the money back tomorrow."

I walked out and spoke with him for a while. It was a really unusual experience and an unusual request to randomly show up at my door that late and ask me for that. I could see his arm was messed up, and I told him, "Okay, I'm going to trust you, but I'm counting on you to come back tomorrow and give me the money back like you said you would." He said, "Oh, for sure, for sure. I will bring you the money back."

The next day, I waited until around 9 or 10 PM, then went to sleep thinking, "Okay, well, he just took the money." About two or three days later, there was a knock on my door around 9 PM. I opened it., "Hey." I asked, "Do you have the money?" He replied, "No, I don't. I'm sorry. Some things happened, and I wanted to come back to you. I really apologize. I know I said I was going to come back." At this point, I was a little angry, not really super angry, but a little bit. He said, "Well, I was wondering if I could borrow another $20 because I still haven't gotten that health card." AT that point I was very upset and said, "No, you said you were going to bring it back. I'm not going to give you more money. You didn't do what you said you would." I went on and on a little bit, and then he looked at me very coldly and said, "Okay. That's too bad because there was someone in front of your house that I wanted you to meet."

In front of my house, there was a big block wall because we had a swimming pool. You had to go out the gate to actually get to the front driveway and sidewalk. After telling me that he had hoped I would qualify to be introduced to this friend of his, he left, leaving a big question in my mind about what that was all about.

Later on, as my yoga practice progressed, I would wake up in the middle of the night and look out the window next to my bed for no reason. I would look out into a part of the sky where there were no stars and blankly stare until a star would finally appear. This started happening a lot for a couple of weeks. I would wake up every night or so, look out, and see this weird experience. As I practiced my physical yoga and balanced on one foot, I would pick one spot on the wall to focus on. I focused and focused until it became so ingrained in my mind that I could sit and relax anywhere, and always be able to focus on a spot which was always conveniently in the center of my vision. Eventually, that spot became a sparkle of light, a candle flame, or a reflection of something always straight and cantered in my vision, wherever I happened to rest, standing or sitting. After that, stars started appearing.

During this time, I drove out to Sedona, Arizona, from Las Vegas. We stopped at Pat Tempe hot springs in Utah and stayed at a friend's house in Hurricane, Utah. They were an older group of people, more middle-aged. Towards the end of the evening, I took some space and went to the front of the house. I looked out into the sky across the horizon and purposely found a space where there were no stars to see what would happen if I just blankly stared. Sure enough, a bright star appeared which startled me. I looked straight up, thinking another bright star would appear, but instead, a brilliant, bright red light swooped from the horizon, circled, and ended up above me. Another light came from behind me, doing the same thing, making an arc, circling, and then stopping above. At that point, I was kind of startled and unsure what was going on. I looked to my right and saw what I thought were a couple of stars moving. Then a movement to my left caught my attention. I turned and looked up, and there was a giant sphere of light that came out of the sky and "landed" behind the house.

I went through the house to the back and knocked on the door of Tom, the person who owned the house. His bedroom door opened to the backyard. I knocked and knocked, saying, "Tom, can I talk to you?" He replied in a very harsh and unusual voice, "No, I'm busy." I thought that was kind of weird, so I went to the front of the house and ended up sleeping on the driveway. In the morning, there was no sign of anything in the backyard. We drove that morning to the rest of our trip to Sedona. As soon as we got there, the driver set up his tent and went to sleep. I went into the bushes to pee, and as I was finishing, a locust came flying out of nowhere and hit me right between my eyebrows. When that happened, I suddenly heard a loud humming, buzzing sound. I looked up to see where it was coming from because it was coming from the sky. I saw a large light, the same red-amberish light, moving from my right side toward the centre of my vision as I looked up into the sky. When it got to the centre, it stopped, the sound stopped, and then it continued, making the sound again as it moved at a right angle away from me. These experiences always affirmed that things weren't as they appeared. I began to become keenly aware of honesty as began leaving my job as a private investigator with my father and begin to focus more on my study of medicine. As you might guess, I didn't tell many people of these experiences.

I don't know to what depth Gavin has had those experiences, but I do know that my older sister Belinda and my father had some very unusual experiences of being held down or "operated" on by strange "spirit" beings. My father, I, my older sister Belinda, and my older sister Christy all have the same look, the same shape of eyes, and a similar look with our hair, eyes, and eyebrows, similar to our great-aunt, my father's aunt, who was a mystic. And so I've never asked, but I wonder sometimes if Gavin has ever had these kinds of experiences.

There is another experience I had in the house where I woke up, and right above my body, about two feet above, was some kind of creature with a bird-like face. It screamed and then somehow popped into another dimension. When I was younger, I had even more bizarre experiences. The earliest memory I have is floating in a box, like floating in a big giant box of windows or a box of glass where you could see the outside. On the outside, we could see the Earth at a distance or below us, and the people with me were all babies. We would be floating past each other, looking at each other, unable to talk, but kind of weightless and floating around in this box. That's my earliest memory.

The next earliest memory I have is standing by a bucket, and I know this because the bucket came up to my shoulders, so I was very, very little. I went to the nearby bedroom where I had a special doll that I used to carry around all the time named Bobby. I went to the lower shelf, placed Bobby on it, and he started shaking back and forth, trembling, and then split into two dolls. I had a hard time understanding that because I had never seen anything like it. So I reached out with both hands and picked up both dolls, one in each hand, touching and seeing them. I could tell for sure that they were real. I put them back on the shelf, and they both shook and then snapped together to make one doll again. I left the room to find my mother to tell her what I had just experienced, but I couldn't speak. I didn't have any words to convey it to her, although I've remembered the full event ever since it happened. But at the time, I did not know how to speak. These types of phenomena were prevalent in my family and created a certain level of stress, at least for my sister and myself. I don't believe that my brothers Hal or Brian ever had these experiences, but they really influenced us and always fascinated us.

In our house, the level of creativity, passion, emotion, and curiosity was very extreme in my childhood. Hyper impressions and ideas were constantly with us. Perhaps this added to some of the "extra-terrestrial" events my father and sister Belinda experienced. I remember having experiences that led me to keep a pillow on my head while I slept. When asked about this, I would always say that I hoped to confuse the pillow-headed people when they came in, so they wouldn't take me, thinking I was one of them. Many years later I saw Whitley Striker's movie Contact and they used those words "pillow headed." A few years after that, in a hypnotic age regression, I remembered being taken up into a craft and having a probe put into the back of my head while a strong-looking person tried to keep my attention. Because I was difficult and not willing to cooperate, I was let down from the metal railing of the craft/room above the house and back into my bedroom.

When The X-Files came out, I sometimes half-joked that it was about my brother Gavin because the events were so weird. As far as I knew (I never asked), Gavin was part of the secret service.

When I was about 7 years old, a Yogi from India began hanging out at our house and cooked food for us once in a while. My mother and father became regular yoga practitioners, fasting occasionally and becoming vegetarians. My father was doing advanced body cleanses, such as putting a string into his nose and pulling it out through his mouth, back and forth. His nostrils became sensitive and clean, and he became known for having a keen sense of smell.

Thanks to my father who had matched the money I had saved, I had the good fortune to go to Himalayas in India when I was 22, and unexpectedly met Babaji, who saved the lives of the two older women I was traveling with, and myself. Because of his mysterious appearing and disappearing, we were saved from the massive earthquake that killed hundreds and left thousands homeless in 1991. The epicenter was in Gangotri, India, the place where we would have been had Babaji not appeared, encouraging us to change our intended destination. So we found someone who thought they knew this Babaji that had appeared to us, and where he might possibly live. We spent many hours driving and hiking through the mountains, until we found him. A couple days after we found him, the 6.3 earthquake happened. After the earthquake he walked up to me. I was standing on a hill, and admiring the beautiful spread of the magical valley in front of me. Babaji came walking up to me and looking at me he lifted his hands up in the air. I responded to him. Babaji was practicing strict silence at the time and would only write on a little chalkboard he carried if he really needed to communicated something that people didn't get from his gestures. This went back and forth with us lifting our hands and then putting them down, several times. And then like an explosion we both just started laughing and laughing and laughing. I was bent over and stood up wiping the tears out of my eyes. I looked over at him and where his head had been was now just a ball of light. His head was completely gone, it was JUST LIGHT. I had had many unusual experiences in my life but this one really impacted me. However the most magical experience of my life would probably be when my great grandmother Maria came to visit my family and stay with us. I would sit on her lap as she would pray over her rosary beads and cry. She was a Mexican woman and her family had everything when she was young, and having lost everything in the Mexican revolution she became focussed on family and the spiritual. Those moments sitting on her lap were the sweetest experiences of my life.

When I first met with Gavin at his home in Fiji, with his 12 kids, I was also introduced to his gardener. Interestingly, the gardener had a place that looked like a temazcal, a solid sweat lodge resembling a low-ceiling igloo. He looked like he was from India, and in front of this structure was a trident set in the way you would find in India with holy men. I was speechless, which seems to be a very common reaction I had when spending time with him when I was younger and only now am beginning to communicate more.

In Gavin's personal quarters there in Fiji was one picture, an artist's rendering of Babaji. Again, I was speechless. This was about 12 years after my meeting with Babaji in the Himalayas, so I really did not know what to say. Years later, I would ask him, and he would tell me that it was symbolic of things he valued.

Later I would take my family to go see Babaji. We stopped in Rome where we got our visas for India. It was 22 years after meeting Babaji the first time, and I thought it would be an amazing time since the Sun "breathes" or fully cycles in and out every 22 years in an expanding and contracting cycle. While we were waiting there was a massive flood that wiped out the area I was going to take the kids to. The magical story of what happened in that flood was covered in a movie. In this area is an ancient temple that is at least 5,000 years old. Just as the waters came rushing down, suddenly wiping out everyone in that village of Kedarnath, a gigantic boulder fell from the mountainside and stopped rolling right behind the temple, a moment before the water came to carry the temple away in its harsh sweep through the valley. Because of the boulder, the water hit the boulder which deflected the water to rush around the temple instead of right through it.

CHAPTER 9

AUTHORITY

In every way, shape, and form, Gavin has been anti-authority. He has said in a dozen ways how he values the sense of knowing. The kind that comes to us when the discomfort in our belly signals the necessity to go to the toilet. The wealthy have a natural sense of authority and understand that few have the authority that is wielded with big guns, big bank accounts, and big stocks of resources. However, in my opinion, the authority that Gavin speaks of is through receiving advice that has not been scrutinized.

There are different kinds of authority: from inheritance, from tradition, and as explained from the German Sociologist, known for his "Protestant ethic",

Max Weber, who defined traditional authority as based on sources of power and leadership styles. Traditional authority is when a person receives their decision-making power through long-standing customs, traditions, or lineage. Power comes from people's acceptance of its validity over time. There is also charismatic and bureaucratic authority, or legal authority, which is based on the position or office someone holds.

Traditional authority can be inherited or seized through brute force or through religious custom. This type of authority provides clarity and ease of transfer, helping to ensure the continuation of culture and tradition. Like a monarchy, it can be very beneficial to the people and society if the rulers are good and trusted friends of the society. However, this type of authority is very difficult to end if the rulers no longer serve the greatest good of the people. Another downside is that the ruler may not actually be qualified in the traditional sense of the word or have helpful skills. Long-term ruling in authority can lead to laws that serve only the group the authority feels aligned with, which might be a very small group of people.

In the intricate and sophisticated culture of Bali, there is a secret mapping of leadership that became known to the general public only in the last few decades. The leader was one who maintained a cosmology where everyone was considered equal. Leaders would come together to discuss bigger plans for collective effort and use of resources. But in general, their reign was over a small number of homes, families, and a small community. Based on the relationship of an individual's birth with the tide, a kind of biorhythm was created, and that "calendar" would have three different kinds of days.

One day is used to plan a presentation, idea, or direction, command, or just instigate more curiosity and consideration, starting the conversation — the planning day. The next day is for the presentation, inception, or just the initiation of a discussion, which might or might not lead to an action. Being prepared for the day when the highest scope of perception was achieved is very important.

I find it interesting that I have to consistently correct my writing when I write about ancient cultures. I automatically write as if in past tense, and then almost immediately I have to correct it because it is present tense. This is one of the most significant facts of ancient traditions and medical systems: they were functional enough to still produce healthy, happy people. Some cultures have easily integrated with the modern world without losing much of their culture. Other cultures were completely absorbed into modern imperialism, and still others went into hiding and retreated deeper into harder-to-reach areas to maintain their knowledge and cosmology, which gave them great meaning and a certain level of access to a kind of magic that is definitely perceived when crossing their path.

Bali is one of the only places where the diverse culture was completely unaffected by the encroachment of modern and foreign cultures, at least until quite recently. One reason that is considered a major factor is because they utilized this day system/calendar to establish who would lead a community into consideration. During the day when an individual was placed in the spotlight, regardless of ability, leadership skills, academic background, or personality type, the rest of the small community would recognize that this day allowed the person to see clearly (perhaps clearer than anyone else because of their "elevation") and have tremendous energy to wield their plan. The community would encourage that person to initiate any kind of discussion or even a specific plan. Doing this always gave each member the opportunity to shine as much as they could, be seen, and be heard.

Our own sense of knowing allows us to take what we have experienced and qualify it, to determine if the information we receive is valid or helpful for us. This is an important idea because so much information is coming at us from many directions. We can get feeds on the current condition of the world without asking, and then others who have received the same, similar, or even different information can bring it to us. Discovering an honest source of information is an on-going process. What will actually help us is up to us to know. We rely too much on external information and expect other people with greater authority to take care of us and protect us. This is not the correct view if we want to be protected from danger and not waste time running after things that give no value or protection to our life.

CHAPTER 10

HEALTH

So what is health? Is this really a question to ask someone else? The ability to be flexible and strong, to sleep well, to make the choices to enjoy what we love, to not be in pain, and to not get physically ill without the bodies' ability to respond appropriately—these are all qualities of health that I consider. These are also very much part of the perspective indigenous traditional medicine, along with the qualities of kindness, generosity, compassion, patience, and concentration - happiness - mental health. Being able to have the strength, energy and capacity and integrate the stressful experiences of life is health.

Getting sick is considered a part of your body's ability to fight an illness. If your body cannot throw up, have diarrhea, or get feverish, then it's an indication of a lack of health. This may surprise some. The cause of ill health, as stated through Tibetan Medicine and in general the sum total of Middle Eastern and Asian indigenous medicine thinking, is the forgetfulness of two things: "The two things are: Forgetfulness that everything changes; and forgetfulness that nothing is disconnected from anything anywhere. An independent existence is a projected idea when looking at the totality of life. Because the temporary and non-independent nature of everything is forgotten, we react emotionally, which leads us into actions and choices that result in dis-harmony." This results in what is called "diseases from natural causes." Traditionally, there are also diseases caused from accidents(like the third leading cause of death in the United States), poisoning(like from pesticides, experimental food, and poisonous medicines like vaccinations), bad energy, and paying for bad actions done in the past("Karmic disease)".

From this definition, hopefully one could understand that in a non-traditional modern culture, addressing disconnection, relationships, and emotions would become a major study for anyone interested in health. How to proceed with interactions that would instill these basic support systems is what I have seen as being a certain kind of victory for Gavin. He is interested in taking good care of his physical body, but I would say that I don't get the impression that bio hacking, supplement wizardry, or dietary hyper-focus rules his day or builds the path into his world. My experience is that even his own health challenges are considered slowly and wisely, without rushing into just whatever information happens to come across his desk with promises of everlasting life. As I contemplated writing the book this way, I understood I had to rely on what my experience was of him and the conversations we had. And at least some of what my brother's secrets were for being so healthy were evident expressions of what has worked for thousands of years.

The main qualities that stood out are **self-reliance**. My brother Gavin is completely self-reliant. He lives on a farm in the middle of nowhere, he hardly sees doctors, never uses pharmaceutical drugs, and doesn't go to hospitals. The next secret is honesty. He always tells you exactly what he's thinking, and you can be sure that if you're talking with him, he's going to tell you honestly how he feels. The third secret is humor. He's a very humorous and sarcastic person and doesn't take himself too seriously, which is exceptional given the scope of stress and seriousness he deals with every day in his work.

The fourth secret is **courage**. My brother always has the courage to think independently. He's not influenced by external information or by figures of authority. And the fifth secret is **family**. Family is his pastime. You can be sure that if he's not working, he's spending quality time in the presence of his family.

Along with a few other qualities, I believe these factors have contributed most to my brother's health and well-being. They are most impactful in developing a character that can withstand the pushback of clarity and direction. Many readers may be searching for a secret drug, an exclusively expensive supplement, or a magical therapy that only the elite have access to. I've done my best in my studies, work and practice, to highlight those things which for thousands of years have been contributing factors to good health and long life. Negative emotions that damage our self-image and confuse our meaning and purpose in life have always been recommended as something that can have a purpose in life but only with caution and awareness so that the naturally damaging effects do not destroy whatever benefit they might bring to one's life. Relationships, continue to be one of the most influential factors in thriving health and longevity, no matter what the medicine or therapy that one may have access to.

The impact of medicine will be affected by the negative or positive influences that one exposes themselves to and that one nourishes inside oneself as they relate to themselves and the world around them. Often the access itself is limited by wrong relationships and unresolved habits of perception and communication that destroy the clarity in choosing, administering, and receiving correct substances that could help us. In the same way, our responses to our emotions and the changes of the seasons, the changes of our age and activities—if we respond in a less than optimal way, we will get less than optimal results from the medicine and benefit that all of that has to offer us.

As I sat in my life and family, curious about my older brother and older sister, I realized over time that my imagination created a preconception that subtly impacted how I would feel about reaching out to him and how I would be thinking and perceiving his responses. As I've gotten to know him better, I realized that much of my self-generated preconceptions were influenced by my own relations with my brothers and sisters or with my father and mother. I remember a story of my younger brother, who reached out to Gavin for some financial help due to a bad decision my younger brother unintentionally made in purchasing a home that had hidden issues costing a lot of money to repair. Gavin wrote back to my brother and told him about the money. The answer was no. Often the most important things we don't really notice until we're about to lose them. About the most important things, we think least, such as our breath. We hear this every day.

Today in this world, for a person who has the ability to go where they want, do what they want, influence programs and projects, implement ideas and personal agendas, a long life is, of course, a much more valuable commodity to them than to many other people who do not have that same kind of freedom in the world.

Although they may be able to buy research labs and develop special supplements and therapies to renew and rejuvenate their body, there is much more to resource. Through the unbroken inquiry of medical and mystical geniuses, over thousands of years, it was discovered that a long, thriving, and healthy life could definitely be established through self-improvement, self-gain, and mastery over one's heart and mind, bringing the natural elements, and even mythologically speaking, the gods and demigods themselves, to the beckoning of one so powerful and focused. However, in the ancient epics, it was also shown that even the richest and most powerful, in the end, had to come to terms with their unquenchable thirst for more power, more riches, more stimulation. In their demanding for more respect, and more acknowledgment from the rest of the universe, damage to themself would occur, to their loved ones, and to all of the natural beauty of the world, poisoning the environment and manipulating everyone to serve only the longevity of the antagonist.

It's well known that some of the men and women who have had the most impact on this world have had very little for themselves. They weren't necessarily the greatest kings, queens, emperors, and empresses. Many of them had very little. There's an amusing story where a great mystic impacted one of the most powerful kings in history by a few words and ideas. The king, in all of his sincerity, offered the entire kingdom to this mystic for giving him a gift so valuable that even with all his riches, he could have never bought. The sage smiled kindly and thanked the king, asking if now the king would take care of the sage's new kingdom for him. In ancient traditional indigenous medicine, our connection or relationship to life itself is always changing until the day we die. And even then, our body transforms either into light or the elements that are compounded to form our body. The body's ability to respond to what is happening in those changes is intrinsically connected to the health of the relationships that we are establishing every moment through our choice to respond in specific ways.

Those responses were mapped out by ancient sages and geniuses of medicine so that we could enhance the intelligence of how the body responds and how the body learns and improves in its own ability to translate the impressions and produce a response that creates more harmony, ease, and effortless choice and change towards life. Knowing this, many encouraged proper relations with family and community nature and mapped out a way to support a long and healthy life. Ignoring that wisdom and valuing the pursuit of certain preferences that sacrificed good relationships created a culture that completely abandoned thousands of years of wisdom that would help guide cultures into healthy and happy long lives that still exist today.

There are dozens of cultures that learned how to avoid serious illness, mitigate minor imbalances, promote stronger genetics, and enhance their life with beauty on many levels within their culture: music, architecture, textiles, dance, song and philosophy. Many of these cultures still have the fruit of the hard work of hundreds of generations.

Now, in an effort to survive the modern attitude of consumption without consideration, they have struggled and have had a great loss in both tradition and culture in their efforts to respond to a new idea of authority without discrimination. There are over 1,700 billionaires in the world today, each having their own story and history. Inheriting values and ideas often established by authority in their efforts to experience more health and develop expensive medicines and therapies, which are soon replaced by new experiments and new efforts. The trillions of dollars that are spent trying to unlock the secret of life unfortunately consistently miss the target in an effort to rewrite the book of life that took thousands of years to translate into understanding how to live as a human where nature itself supports the strength and intelligence of the body to live long and thrive.

As a wise man once said, "You can't fix stupid."